2018

Aloe Vera Nature's Little Secret

WRITTEN BY

MARIA D. TALTON

Table of Content

WHAT IS ALOE VERA?

You most likely know aloe has been utilized for a considerable length of time to treat consumers and burns. It's most likely safe to state, you've even utilized it for no less than one of those two. Is it accurate to say that you are mindful that aloe is alluded to by numerous scientists as "Nature's Miracle" as a result of lots of different afflictions it can treat? Odds are you didn't.

That is on account of the huge medication organizations don't need you to think about that.

They have held it under wraps since they profit through research of ailment treating drugs. It takes years and a huge number of dollars to discover a medication, test it, and lastly showcase it. That at that point supports their next undertaking. It's an atrocious cycle that never closes.

The medication organizations don't have sufficient energy (or essentially would prefer not to) to consider the advantages of normal medicines, cures, and antidotes. There is no cash to be produced using anything that can't be protected. Shockingly for every one of us, they are a business and cash is all that really matters.

Is Aloe Vera extremely a supernatural existence plant? Numerous realities and proceeded with inspecting are available, so you may choose for yourself. Sorted out pharmaceutical and pharmacology have not seized Aloe since it can't be licensed and its utilization weakens actually several remedies and non-doctor prescribed medications. Aloe Vera is hypoallergenic and has no known symptoms even in extensive measurements."

As a succulent, Aloe Vera is a prickly plant. Its thick, plump leaves store water and its underlying foundations become evenly close to the surface of the dirt to get the little water that exists where it thrives– primarily in the hot, dry deserts of Africa. Tubular yellow blossoms become out of the Aloe Vera, bringing about it being expelled from its regular living space for family unit enhancement. Be that as it may, Aloe Vera isn't just prevalent in the home for its delightful appearance. Inside its long, tubular leaves, which become out of bubbles, is a dreary aloe gel that has picked up huge respect in the society for its numerous restorative properties.

Aloe Vera is turning into a trailblazer in elective medication, giving a characteristic alternative to numerous people hoping to recover their safety burdens or secure their general comfort. Long being suspected for its medical advantages, aloe Vera shows up in stone carvings from Egypt dated 6,000 years earlier. Since aloe was covered with pharaohs as a present for existence in the wake of death, the Egyptians nicknamed this plant the "plant of immortality"– and they may have hit the nail on the head, as late research affirms aloe's capacity to battle and avoid numerous diseases, in this manner possibly giving us the award of a more drawn out, more beneficial life.

HISTORY OF ALOE VERA

EGYPT:

The fundamental known report gives an account of the supporting juice of the Aloe Vera plant reaches as far back as 6,000 years earlier in old Egypt. Aloe was seen as a holy plant the "blood" of which held the way to heavenliness, prosperity, and everlasting status. Both Cleopatra and Nefertiti inexplicably regarded the maintaining juice and used it as a bit of their step by step skin and brilliance of mind. The utilization of aloe was seen as the journey for physical gloriousness. To be sure, even the dead were protected with Aloe Vera by virtue of its unfriendly to bacterial and against developments attributes. The fundamental conviction was that in stopping the physical breaking down process everlasting life could be proficient – both on a physical and a supernatural level. Aloe was known as the "plant of until the end of time". Its moderating and misery reducing sway were accounted for in the "papyrus Eber" of 1,550 BC.

MESOPOTAMIA:

The most prompt documentation of Aloe was found on the mud sheets from Nippur which retreat as long earlier as 2,200 BC. The overall public of this time was by then aware of the refining effect of aloe on the assimilation tracts, in this season of history illnesses were continually seen as a shrewd responsibility for body and only an amazing plant, for instance, aloe had the trademark energy to expel the fallen angels.

ALEXANDER THE GREAT:

In the periods of Alexander, the Great Aloe Vera was consistently used for restorative treatment in the countries of Asia. It is recorded that Alexander the Great used the use of aloe juice to recover the war wounds to his warriors (356 - 323 B.C.)

Alexander went to the level of having transportable trucks of planted Aloe for sensible reasons with a particular ultimate objective to have new supplies ready for action in the midst of his different battle campaigns. It is expressed, that Aristotle convinced Alexander the Great to get the Island Socotra especially to get responsibility for gainful aloe sticks – in doing all things considered Alexander acquired satisfactory pharmaceutical to recover the wounds of his entire units.

DIOSKURIDES:

Further bolstering their good fortune the Romans took after the smartness of the Egyptians and Greeks by in like manner using the repairing powers of the Aloe Vera plant. In the middle of the reign of Emperor Nero in around 50 B.C., the specialist and naturalist Dioscorides wandered the whole of the orient asking about new systems for the arrangement. He formed a couple of books training on pharmaceutics which incorporated various pharmaceuticals for the treatment of boundless diseases.

In his wide areas in perspective of the valuable results of plant treatment, he shows the aloe as one of his most cherished recovering plants. He recommended the use of aloe juice for the different physical issue, for instance, the treatment of wounds, stomach upsets, gingivitis, arthralgia, skin aggravation, sunburn, skin irritation, male example hair sparseness, et cetera.

CHINESE MEDICINE:

In Chinese culture, aloe has been a vital fixing in restorative medicines since the seasons of the Marco Polo actions. The treatment book of Shi-Shen portrayed aloe Vera as the "Strategy for Harmony"- the plant expected a remarkable part of the regular day to day existence of the Chinese.

The Japanese culture additionally enormously values the aloe plant, in Japan, it was known as the "illustrious plant", the juice was expended as a mixture and the samurai utilized it for medicinal liquid that is rubbed into the skin to relieve muscular stiffness and pain.

COLUMBUS:

New universes were found with the guide of Aloe Vera, Christopher Columbus was known to have aloe Vera creating in plant pots on his feet of watercraft and the plant was used to repair the wounds of his employed runners.

In the middle of the sixteenth century, Spanish Jesuit clerics - obtained the wild aloe Vera and were known to spread the plant it in districts where it had not yet been produced. Today these clerics are up 'til now celebrated likewise showed philologists and healers. The Maya Indians started the significantly inventive juice of this desert plant as the "Fountain of Youth".

SANSKRIT:

In Sanskrit, aloe is known as Ghrita-Kumari. Kumar concludes young woman and it was assumed that this plant gave the imperativeness of youth to women and had a regenerating power on the female nature.

In the Indian medicate, aloe is associated in different applications, for instance, reestablishing cures, for menorrhea issues and to offset the cardiovascular structure.

ANTHROPOSOPHIC MEDICINE:

As indicated by Rudolf Steiner, the aloe speaks to the moon in trouble with the sun – identifying with the high fluid substance of the plant. A principle trademark is a strain between the ethereal and the astral. An extraordinary aspect of the aloe plant is its capacity to sort out the water, to keep up life and to repeat (various branches!) in desperate conditions: warm, wind, dryness. Because of its hearty external layer and its crowd webbed inward vein framework the aloe figures out how to keep up its dampness by anticipating vanishing; it is a really wonderful survivor of nature.

PRIEST KNEIPP:

Minister Kneipp was an extraordinary admirer of the aloe Vera, in both plant and powder frame. Kneipp was overwhelmingly persuaded of the cleansing and purifying impact on the stomach related framework. The digestive tract and the digestive system related untouchable framework assumed a noteworthy part in the medicines of Kneipp. It is additionally revealed that Kneipp had extraordinary improving achievement while applying the aloe to both infective and degenerative infirmities of the eye.

BENEFITS OF ALOE VERA FOR SKIN

Since we have a decent comprehension of why Aloe Vera is consistently looked for after and utilized, we can start to research a portion of the ways this valuable plant can support and care for our skin.

WOUND HEALING:

Aloe Vera is commonly used as a trademark answer for help with the recovering of wounds like scratches, cuts and expands. The relieving and threatening to bacterial properties help to clean and sterilize wounds, which may support the general recovering procedure.

An examination in 1995 would have liked to study the sufficiency of Aloe Vera in the treatment of consumers. The analysts used a case of 27 individuals, 9 females, and 18 folks, who had been admitted to the consuming unit of Ramathibodi Hospital in Thailand.

The consumed zone was isolated into two proportional estimated regions, with one being treated with a Vaseline dressing treatment and the other with an Aloe Vera course of action. The dressings were cleaned two times each day and the consumers were explored at set up breaks all through the traverse of the examination. The results checked that "the aloe Vera gel-treated sore recovered speedier than the Vaseline fabric district. The typical time of patching in the aloe gel zone was 11.89 days and 18.19 days for the Vaseline material treated damage."

Aloe Vera is furthermore noticeably used to help recover sunburn. Right, when our skin is introduced to viable brilliant pillars from the sun for an extremely lengthy timespan, at last, the skin cells may begin to fail miserably, which triggers a moderating response in your body to help recover and shield the skin from furthermore hurt. The recovering properties of Aloe Vera can be mishandled to help reduce provoke irritation or burden caused by devours, and furthermore to progress and possibly revive the general patching process.

IT ACTS AS A MOISTURIZER:

Aloe saturates the skin without giving it an oily vibe, so it`s ideal for anybody with a slick skin appearance. For ladies who utilize mineral-based makeup, Aloe Vera goes about as a cream and is incredible for the face before the application to counteracts skin drying. For men: Aloe Vera gel can be utilized as a face ointment treatment as its mending properties can treat little cuts caused by shaving.

IT HELPS IN INGESTION:

The inward advantages of Aloe Vera should be similar as stunning. The plant is said to enhance the absorption and to alleviate ulcers. A few people think of it as a purgative, while others ascribe that impact to its stomach related characteristics (which standardize the framework and actuate normality). The juice is additionally endorsed for joint inflammation and ailment. To test any of these cases, soak the cut foliage in water or bite bits of the new leaf.

IT LESSENS THE VISIBILITY OF STRETCH MARKS:

The skin resembles one major bit of versatile that'll extend and contract as expected to suit development. In any case, if the skin extends too far, too quickly (because of pregnancy, fast weight pick up or misfortune) the versatility of the skin can be harmed. That is the thing that leaves those unattractive extend marks. These imprints show up because of minor tears in the layers of the skin caused by sudden and over the top extending. Aloe Vera gel can help conceal these extend checks by recuperating these injuries.

SOOTHES AND HYDRATES:

In perspective of the dry air, Aloe Vera is neighborhood too, its leaves can store huge measures of water to shield the plant from drying out in even the most excellent warms and conditions. Because of this limit, the gel contained inside the leaves is every now and again used as the purpose behind pharmaceutical things proposed to help either hydrate or immerse your skin.

Numerous people ignore that the skin is an organ and that it accepts an uncommonly basic part in ensuring that no harmful toxic substances, chemicals, microorganisms or other outside contaminants progress into your body. Regardless, in light of the way that there are no tremendous wounds doesn't suggest that your skin needn't bother with consistent help to help fend off the bacterial intrusion it faces once every day.

In case your skin isn't honestly hydrated then individual skin cells may begin to pass on and chip. Go skin will most likely end away abraded, which could influence it to end up being considerably less requesting to tear, tear or shape into a rash. By using an aloe Vera-based gel or cream, you may have the ability to ensure that your skin remains hydrated and clean continually, especially in delicate or helpless districts, for instance, around the face and eyes.

ANTIOXIDANT PROPERTIES:

Aloe Vera is a sensational source of vitamins C and E, which are admired for their ability to help shield your body against potential harm from free radical particles.

Free radicals are various to various particles since they have an uneven number of electrons. Electrons are regularly fused and accept an essential part in ensuring that particles are fundamentally tireless. Right when free radical particles associate with your skin cells, they may try and take electrons to outline a relentless match. The mischief caused by this system, called oxidative weight, can break or impact skin cells, which could add to an incapacitated safe structure.

A current report coordinated in China wanted to separate the disease counteractive action operator properties of different developed cases of aloe Vera evacuate against other plant-based blends like Butylated Hydroxytoluene (BHT), a characteristic compound with cell fortification properties, and α-tocopherol, a piece of vitamin E. The examination assumed that "all the aloe isolates demonstrated imperative malignancy counteractive action operator activity" and that "the three-year-old focus demonstrated the most grounded radical seeking development."

There is an extensive variety of Aloe Vera skin creams open that may have the ability to help shield your skin from free radical iotas. Regardless, for the best results, you should need to consider looking for specific creams that have been animated with additional vitamin E, which may improve the quality and profitability of the cream or gel.

TREATMENTS OF SPOTS AND ACNE:

Acne is a skin ailment that is caused when pores on your body end up hampered with dead cells, harms or possibly microorganisms. These zones can begin to show reactions like obstructed pores, whiteheads, spots and even smooth skin.

Aloe Vera, given its unfriendly to microbial properties, is much of the time used as a facial normal answer for help retouch flaws and scars that may be made in light of acne. Aloe Vera is a rich normal wellspring of vitamin C, which can help with the age of collagen, a basic protein that can be found in the skin and other connective tissues. Collagen ensures that skin cells remain supple, firm and strong, which, in the event that you're planning to help fight spots and skin irritation, may be an important extension to your skincare treatment.

A test in 2004 planned to consider the effects of Aloe Vera gel and basic oils on skin break out. 84 student school understudies with skin aggravation were used as the illustration and were disconnected into seven one of a kind social affairs, each one being treated with the other game plan, which was associated two times each day in the wake of washing toward the start of the day and night. The number of wounds was checked toward the beginning of the test, and after that step by step all through the four-week traverse of the examination.

The outcomes of the examination demonstrated that "the sufficiency of the Ocimum oil cream things extended with growing aloe gel substance. Things arranged with the undiluted or half aloe gels were most unique and settled blazing wounds speedier than the standard thing."

ANTI-AGEING BENEFITS:

This last potential advantage aloe Vera may give incorporates a great part of an indistinguishable science from the beforehand talked about subject. Aloe Vera might have the capacity to help advance the generation of collagen to enable keep to skin solid. Without adequate collagen, you may start to see your skin hang, wrinkle and age speedier.

Aloe Vera skin creams, gels, and supplements may have the capacity to help counter these distinctive dermal issues as a result of the various nourishing substance they have. Like we discussed before, vitamin C specifically is known to assume a part in collagen generation, so expanding your admission of this supplement through the utilization or ingestion of Aloe Vera items or supplements might be a perfect answer for help support hostile to maturing endeavors.

Gratefully, there is an extensive variety of various pharmaceutical and excellence items accessible that might have the capacity to help. When searching for the perfect alternative for you, attempt to discover liquor free assortments with a high level of aloe Vera extricate, in light of the fact that they might probably offer better outcomes. You can likewise synchronize these items with your eating regimen by including nourishments like tomatoes, avocados, and nuts with an end goal to augment your admission of accommodating vitamins, minerals, and supplements that may additionally elevate hostile to maturing endeavors to profit your skin.

IT SOOTHES IN PERIODONTAL DISEASE:

As indicated by an examination distributed in the Journal of Ethno pharmacology, it's amazingly useful in the treatment of gum infections like gingivitis, periodontitis. It lessens dying, aggravation and swelling of the gums. It is an intense sterile in pockets where ordinary cleaning is troublesome, and its antifungal properties help extraordinarily in the issue of denture stomatitis, pathos ulcers, broke and split corners of the mouth.

HOW ALOE VERA CAN HELP ECZEMA

Hydrates the skin:

There is great logical confirmation that Aloe Vera gel is a viable cream which can expand the water content in the best layer of the skin (the epidermis). This is believed to be because of the high sugar substance of the gel which enables it to go about as a humectant, drawing in and holding water in the epidermis. Expanding the water substance of the skin can diminish the 'tight' feeling of dermatitis.

Reduces infections:

Eczema is regularly irritated by diseases so limiting them can frequently have a major effect on a general skin inflammation side effects. This is particularly valid for youthful kids who are inclined to getting foul and scratching and whose insusceptible frameworks are as yet building up Several investigations have demonstrated that Aloe Vera gel can restrain the multiplication of different strains of Streptococcus microorganisms and Candida Albicans (a yeast).

Quiets the burn:

Various known mitigating substances have been identified in Aloe Vera gel which can help quietly excited skin inflammation and diminish the relentless tingling. It additionally feels extremely cool when connected to have a prompt quieting impact as well.

May allow hydrocortisone to work better:

There means that Aloe Vera gel may upgrade assimilation of hydrocortisone into the skin, which recommends that utilizing Aloe Vera gel in conjunction with solution steroid cream more viable in quieting dermatitis flare-ups than just steroid creams alone. While more research is expected to comprehend and confirm this discovering, Aloe Vera/hydrocortisone cream is as of now accessible in a few sections of the world.

HEALTH BENEFITS OF ALOE VERA

HELPS EASE MENSTRUAL PAIN:

Amid a lady's menstrual cycle, the uterus commonly contracts in pulsatile, difficult design to dispose of an unfertilized egg. This pain can run from minor to crippling from lady to lady, yet what is relatively all inclusive is they want to shock the irritation. One approach to do as such is to utilize an against convulsive that decreases the recurrence of undesirable ripples. Aloe Vera utilization can act by means of this component, decreasing general torment stack.

HELPS TREAT DEHYDRATION:

Over half of the total population of the world experiences perpetual drying out, however, they are unaware. Aloe Vera can help with this, as the plant is thickly water-based, and helps hydrate you superior to water itself. This could be because of the Aloe Vera gel itself, which holds water. Aloe Vera squeeze likewise normally contains potassium and can be contrasted with coconut water for its utility in keeping up blood liquid adjust. Notwithstanding your decision, simply make certain to get enough water every day.

ASSISTS In BODY's DETOXIFICATION PROCESS:

The great water substance of Aloe Vera is ideal for keeping up ideal kidney work, however, did you realize that it additionally helps with the liver's detoxification of waste? Firmly identified with the cucumber in its water content, Aloe Vera juice is rapidly turning into a most loved with regards to detoxifying the liver. The phytonutrients found in Aloe Vera likewise resets liver chemicals which may have turned out to be lifted.

HELPS TREAT CONSTIPATION:

As specified, Aloe Vera is made out of basically water, which makes it perfect to help with here and now, infrequent blockage. This kind of inconsistency is ordinarily because of drying out and makes the body reuse water from reckless into distribution where cells may require it. This water misfortune brings about compacting of filth, so it turns out to be difficult to travel through the colon. Be that as it may, as water allows expanded, water again is designated to squander evacuation and you encounter a typical stool.

HELPS MANAGE DIABETES:

Studies conducted in both human and creature models have stated that aloe Vera utilization can help counterbalance the incessantly abnormal amounts of glucose, from as meager as expending two teaspoons. In spite of the fact that it isn't precisely clear the component behind its activity, it can be incorporated into a characteristic routine for overseeing diabetes.

REDUCES CHOLESTEROL LEVELS:

While much talk is made about cholesterol levels, triglyceride levels are apparently more essential to oversee, aloe Vera lessens triglyceride levels by as much as 30%, and when overcome with an eating routine rich in monounsaturated fats, and general lipid profiles are fundamentally augmented.

MAY HELP REDUCE THE RISK OF CANCER DEVELOPMENT:

It is said that tumor cells can't make due to basic conditions, and is one reason aloe Vera might be helpful. Moreover, aloe Vera shows mitigating properties, which can keep undesirable changes from jumping out at DNA strands.

BACKINGS THE IMMUNE SYSTEM:

Aloe Vera squeeze and gel contains numerous phytonutrients and against oxidant mixes, which help bolster the well-being of your safe framework. Aloe Vera additionally has hostile to microbial properties, to diminish bacterial or viral load upon introduction to such pathogens.

CAN BE USED AS A DENTAL REMEDY:

Aloe Vera gel can be utilized to expel plaque from teeth and to keep the abundance of microorganisms in the mouth. This additionally helps with avoidance of dental caries, diminishes the occurrence of gingivitis, and in conjunction with a chlorhexidine-based mouthwash can frame a compelling oral mouthwash.

DRINKING BENEFITS OF ALOE VERA

IT's A RICH SOURCE OF SALICYLIC ACID:

Salicylic corrosive present in Aloe Vera controls aggravation by hindering the generation of hormone prostaglandins. Salicylic, similar to headache medicine likewise diminishes irritation by devastating microscopic organisms that reason aggravation.

PREVENTS SWELLING OF LIPS:

Its calming property serves to limit the swelling of the lips.

IMPROVES JOINT FLEXIBILITY:

Aloe Vera contains B-sister role which gives help from joint firmness.

HELPS TREAT ANEMIA:

Ghritkumari Saar is effectively utilized as a part of an Ayurvedic readiness known as Kumari Asava, helpful in remedying stomach related and liver issue, paleness, jaundice, and sicknesses identified with bile pipe annoy bladder, among others.

BALANCES HORMONAL PROBLEM:

The juice is frequently utilized as a part of numerous other homegrown tonics vital in curing hormonal issues, and additionally, pancreas and spleen related scatters.

LOADED WITH VITAMINS AND MINERALS:

The juice comes stacked with a group of vitamins, minerals and cancer prevention agents basic for our body. "The main thing that doesn't discover nearness in aloe vera is Vitamin D," shares Dr. Gautam. Aloe vera juice is effectively accessible in the market. You can begin by expending it plain and after that graduate to attempting it with different juices like amla, giloy, tulsi, and karela.

GOOD FOR WEIGHT LOSS:

It has powerful calming and diuretic properties. The calming properties can help keep your framework up and running consistently advancing nourishment assimilation. The juice additionally expands the body's metabolic rate and fat consume off.

Because of its capable mitigating properties, aloe vera juice is likewise, accepted to alleviate and saturates the bothersome scalp and dry hairs. On the off chance that you discover your hair severing effectively and in various spots, at that point, you need to consider including the Aloe Vera squeeze as a feature of your skincare regimen.

It contains intense vitamins and minerals which help increment your hair quality and adds an excellent sparkle to it.

PROMOTES HAIR GROWTH:

Poor hair development is frequently because of obstructed hair follicles by dead skin cells. It contains effective proteolytic catalysts which help dispose of these dead skin cells from the hair follicles and help advance hair development.

POTENT LAXATIVE:

Aloe vera juice is promoted as a kind of scrub. It gets this notoriety since it contains anthroquinine, which is a powerful diuretic. Notwithstanding the stomach agony and outrageous the runs this diuretic may cause, ingesting aloe vera juice may likewise cause malabsorption of supplements and pharmaceutical and loss of electrolytes, particularly potassium. Low potassium levels may prompt an unpredictable pulse, muscle shortcoming and weakness. The runs may likewise build danger of lack of hydration. Other gastrointestinal protests caused by drinking aloe vera juice incorporate sickness and regurgitating.

Reference links

http://www.aloe-yourmiracledoctor.com/

https://www.medicalnewstoday.com/articles/265800.php

https://www.aloe-medical-group.com/en/aloe-vera/history.html

https://www.scratchsleeves.co.uk/aloe-vera-for-eczema-alternative-remedies/

https://www.naturalfoodseries.com/15-surprising-benefits-aloe-vera/

https://food.ndtv.com/health/7-reasons-to-drink-aloe-vera-juice-everyday-1627032/

www.ingramcontent.com/pod-product-compliance
Lightning Source LLC
Chambersburg PA
CBHW051429250726
48655CB00003B/1313